Magda Karina Cruz García
Rosa María Baltazar Téllez
José Arias Rico

Vaccination schedule in children under 5 years of age

Magda Karina Cruz García
Rosa María Baltazar Téllez
José Arias Rico

Vaccination schedule in children under 5 years of age

Autonomous University of the State of Hidalgo

ScienciaScripts

Imprint

Cover image: www.ingimage.com

This book is a translation from the original published under ISBN 978-613-9-44211-9.

Publisher:
Sciencia Scripts
is a trademark of
Dodo Books Indian Ocean Ltd. and OmniScriptum S.R.L publishing group

120 High Road, East Finchley, London, N2 9ED, United Kingdom
Str. Armeneasca 28/1, office 1, Chisinau MD-2012, Republic of Moldova, Europe
Printed at: see last page
ISBN: 978-620-8-34532-7

Presentation

This book discusses the benefits of complying with the national vaccination schedule for children under five years of age; where it is one of the priorities for the health sector in Mexico; taking into account the high morbidity and mortality rate due to immunopreventable diseases; where vaccination is one of the most effective actions for prevention.

Vaccination is one of the most effective public health actions to prevent diseases and an obligation of the state. However, in Mexico there is no certainty about the coverage and timeliness with which vaccines are given to children during their first year of life (every year 2.3 million children are born in Mexico), these figures mean that up to 65.7% of children may not have their complete schedule or have received it late and, therefore, at risk of getting sick. In contrast, the Federal Health Secretariat in Mexico; admits that only 9.3% of children under one year of age are at risk for vaccine-preventable diseases.

The United Nations Children's Fund (UNICEF), an agency of the United Nations (UN) dedicated to promoting the rights of children and adolescents; designed a campaign "100% Vaccinated Children", whose objective is that vaccines reach the most remote communities in the world and can be administered to all children, wherever they are.

This goes hand in hand with the agreement of experts from the Center for Disease Control (CDC).), the main groups of factors or reasons related to the lack of vaccination are grouped in categories such as vaccination system, communication and information, family characteristics, attitudes and knowledge of the parents in such a way that all these factors contribute to the child not having all the vaccines according to his age, reaching the conclusion of a non-compliance with the National Vaccination Schedule.

Nola Pender, nurse author of the Health Promotion Model (HPM), stated that behavior is motivated by the desire to achieve wellness and human potential.), expressed that behavior is motivated by the desire to achieve well-being and human potential; she was interested in creating a nursing model that would provide answers to how people make decisions about their own health care.

Table of Contents

Chapter 1: Introduction

1.1 Introduction

The infant stage in the preschool years when they are between three and five years old, the child is busy learning language, is acquiring a sense of self and greater independence, and is beginning to learn the workings of the physical world, timely vaccination during this stage is critical because it helps provide immunity before children are exposed to diseases that could be fatal. Vaccines are evaluated to ensure that they are safe and effective for administration to children at recommended ages.(1)

Vaccines can prevent diseases, prolong life, and even eradicate plagues that have existed since prehistoric times. The effectiveness of vaccines has been known for decades, yet children in developing countries still die from vaccine-preventable diseases. The United States and its international partners have been working together for more than 30 years to bring the benefits of vaccines to children everywhere.(2)

Immunization prevents diseases, disabilities, and deaths, such as diphtheria, hepatitis B, measles, mumps, pertussis, pneumonia, polio, rotavirus diarrheal diseases, rubella, and tetanus. (3)

Vaccination is one of the most effective public health actions to prevent diseases and an obligation of the state. However, in Mexico there is no certainty about the coverage and timeliness with which vaccines are given to children during their first year of life (2.3 million children are born each year in Mexico), these figures mean that up to 65.7% of children may not have their complete schedule or may have received it late and, therefore, are at risk of falling ill . In contrast, the SSA admits that only 9.3% of children under one year of age are at risk for vaccine-preventable diseases. (3,4)

That is why UNICEF has launched the "100% Vaccinated Children" campaign, which aims to ensure that vaccines reach the world's most remote communities and can be administered to all children, wherever they may be. (4,5)

According to experts from the Center for Disease Control (CDC)), the main groups of factors or reasons related to the lack of vaccination are grouped in categories such as vaccination system, communication and information, family characteristics, attitudes and knowledge of the parents in such a way that all these factors contribute to the child not having all the vaccines according to his age, reaching the conclusion of non-compliance with the National Immunization Schedule. (6-8)

Nola Pender, nurse author of the Health Promotion Model (HPM), stated that behavior is motivated by the desire to achieve wellness and human potential.), expressed that behavior is motivated by the desire to achieve well-being and human potential; she was interested in creating a nursing model that would provide answers to how people make decisions about their own health care. (9) Therefore, it was decided to use individual characteristics and experiences, nutrition, exercise, health responsibility, stress management, interpersonal relationships and self-actualization, with emphasis on the affects related to specific behavior in personal influences and situational influences. (10) The range established by this theorist allows us to link it to the project, analyzing individual characteristics and experiences, relative to specific behavior in personal influences and situational influences on individuals.

1.2 Problem Statement research

The Secretariat of Health of Hidalgo (SSH) urged parents to complete their children's vaccination schedule, since Mexico has increased the protection of the population, especially children under five years of age, with the application of 4 to 8 vaccines that protect against 13 diseases. (15,16)

Among the diseases against which children receive protection through immunization are tuberculosis, measles, rubella, diphtheria, pertussis, tetanus, polio, mumps, hepatitis, influenza, tetanus, severe pneumococcal infection and rotavirus. The SSH specialists emphasized the importance of applying vaccines according to the age of the child, as it represents a protection for them, since the boosters that are applied within the scheme for children under 5 years of age are to increase the memory of antibodies given by the previous doses, and thus expand the defense of children from the risk of suffering from these diseases. (15,17)

As part of this protection scheme that is applied to children under 2, 4, 6 and 18 months of age, there is the Pentavalent and Hexavalent vaccine that protects children against Diphtheria, Tetanus, Pertussis, Influenza type B and Hepatitis B, and to 4 year olds as a booster of the DPT vaccine against Diphtheria, Tetanus and Pertussis. against Diphtheria, Tetanus and Pertussis . (18)

In Hidalgo, different strategies are carried out by the health sector, where in 100% of the units, vaccines are provided according to the age group. In addition, with regular personnel of the SSH, semi-fixed posts are placed with vaccinators to bring the actions at strategic points in places of high concentration in urban areas and rural localities, in addition to the actions carried out during the National Health Weeks.

Currently in Hidalgo, there is a 100% vaccine supply of Pentavalent or Hexavalent vaccine, which includes fractions of the composition of the DPT vaccine. For this reason, the Ministry of Health urged parents to take their children under 5 years of age to the medical units, so that according to the National Health Card, they can complete their vaccination schedule; It is thought that there are factors why mothers do not go to the different vaccination sites with their children, even knowing the benefits that vaccination brings to their children under 5 years old, and many of them lack or even miss the doses of vaccines, they do not have the necessary time, they do not feel sure of what they are administering to their children, some do not have the knowledge of the importance of vaccines, also they are single mothers or do not have a support, they do not have the economy to cover their expenses; They do not have a stable job, thus demonstrating the lack of compliance in the vaccination of their children.(10,19)

Nola Pender's health promotion model illustrates the multifaceted nature of people in their interaction with the environment when trying to achieve the desired state of health; it emphasizes the link between personal influences and situational influences we refer to experiences, knowledge, beliefs; linked to the health behaviors or behaviors that are intended to be achieved, so the following question arises. (9)

1.3 General Objective

To determine the factors that influence non-compliance with the vaccination schedule in children under 5 years of age in a preschool school located in the community of San Juan Tizahuapan, Epazoyucan, Hidalgo.

1.4 Specific objectives

1. To identify the social factors (occupation, age, level of education) involved in non-compliance with the complete vaccination schedule.

2. To recognize the cultural factors (beliefs, myths and truths about vaccination) that affect non-compliance with the vaccination schedule in schoolchildren under 5 years of age.

3. To determine the influence of parental self-discipline on compliance with the National Vaccination Schedule in schoolchildren under 5 years of age.

1.5 Hypotheses

H1:
There are factors that influence non-compliance with the vaccination schedule in children under 5 years of age in a preschool school located in the community of San Juan Tizahuapan, Epazoyucan, Hidalgo.

H0:
There are no factors that influence non-compliance with the vaccination schedule in children under 5 years of age in a preschool school located in the community of San Juan Tizahuapan, Epazoyucan, Hidalgo.

1.6 Theoretical framework

1.6.1 Theoretical Nola Pender

This theory explains the relationships between the factors that influence health behavior. This model relies on education on how people should take care of themselves and try to lead a healthy life.

Graph 1
Nola's general framework Pender.

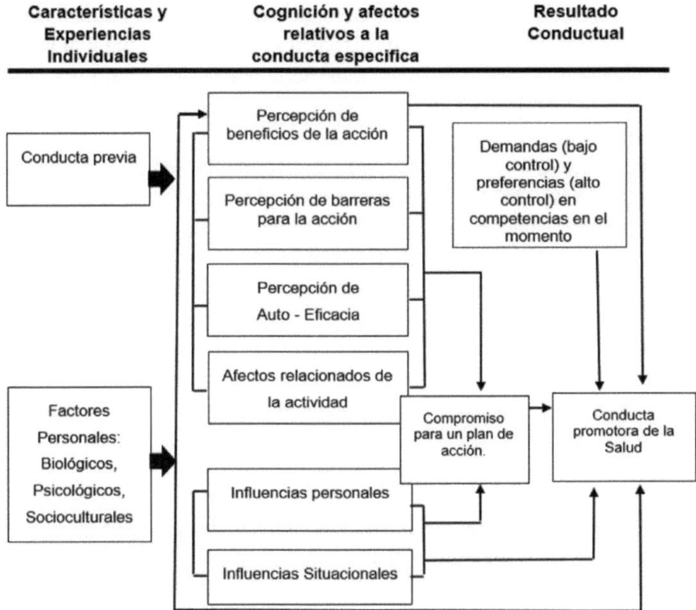

Source: Pender's 1978 model of health promotion. In Cid PH, Merino, JE Stiepovich

Nola Pender stated that "we must promote healthy living, which is more important than care, because in that way there are fewer sick people, fewer resources are spent, people are given independence and the future is improved" (9). (9)

Metaparadigms

Health: He gives great importance to this concept, it is a highly positive state.

Person: Is the individual and the center of the theorist. Each person is unique and unrepeatable and is defined by a pattern of perceptual knowledge and variable factors.

Environment: It is not described with precision, but the interactions between cognitive-preceptual factors and modifying factors that influence the appearance of health-promoting behaviors are represented.

Nursing: The welfare of the nurse has personal responsibility in health care, it is the basis of any reform plan for such citizens and the nurse is the main agent in charge of motivating users to maintain their personal health. (9,62)

Conceptualization

Individual characteristics and experiences, previous related behavior, frequency of the same behavior. Direct and indirect effects of engaging in health-promoting behaviors, personal factors, predictors of certain behavior; previous related behavior: frequency of the same or similar behavior in the past, direct or indirect effects of the likelihood of engaging in health-promoting behaviors.

Personal factors: refers to all factors related to people that influence the individual to relate to his or her environment in order to develop health-promoting behaviors, including biological, psychological and sociocultural factors, in addition to the perceived benefits of health-promoting actions, as well as the barriers he or she encounters to these behaviors.

Situational influences: these are the perceptions and cognitions of any given situation or context that may facilitate or impede behavior.

Cognitive-preceptual factors: these are the primary motivational mechanisms of health promotion activities. (62)

Graph 2

Location of the research problem in the model.

Factores que influyen en el incumplimiento de la vacunación en niños de 3 a 5 años.
Influencias Personales
Influencias Situacionales
Conducta Promotora de la Salud en las Vacunas

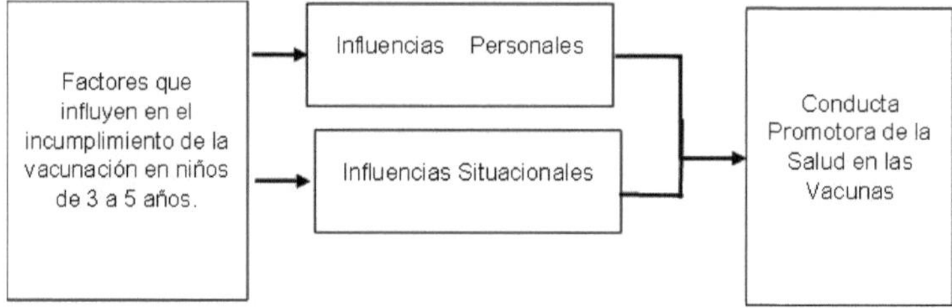

Source: Nola Pender model (2003).

Health care behavior is influenced by personal actions, such as the information we have received about something, and based on situational influences on previous experiences and knowledge.

1.6.2 Vaccine s

A vaccine is a preparation intended to generate acquired immunity against a disease by stimulating the production of antibodies, containing an agent that closely resembles the disease-causing microorganism, which is made from attenuated forms of the microbe, killed microbes modified in safe environments, their toxins or one of their surface proteins. (1) The agent stimulates the body's immune system to recognize the agent as a threat, destroy it and keep a record of it, so that the immune system can more easily recognize and destroy any such microorganisms it encounters later.

Vaccines are used prophylactically, i.e., to prevent or lessen the effects of a future infection by some natural pathogen, the administration of a vaccine is called vaccination. (36)

The vaccination schedule is the chronological sequence of vaccines that are systematically administered to the entire population in a country or geographical area, in order to obtain adequate immunization of the population against diseases for which an effective vaccine is available.
These schedules are modified according to the availability of new vaccines and the evolution of the epidemiological situation of the different vaccine-preventable diseases. The universal vaccination program is a public health policy whose objective is to provide specific protection to the population against vaccine-preventable diseases. (1)

This is aligned with the Political Constitution of the United Mexican States, in addition to the following laws, codes, regulations, decrees and Mexican Official Standards. Mexican Official Standard NOM-004-SSA3-2012, Del Expediente Clínico. DOF 15-10-2012. Official Mexican Standard NOM-047-SSA1-1993 On organic solvents in occupationally exposed personnel. DOF 15-10-2012. Official Mexican Standard NOM-036-SSA2-2012, Prevention and control of diseases. Application of vaccines, toxoids, faboterapics (sera) and immunoglobulins in humans. DOF 28-09-2012. Norma Oficial Mexicana NOM-017-SSA2-2012, For epidemiological surveillance. DOF 19-02-2013.

Mexican Official Standard NOM-087-SEMARNAT SSA1-2002. Biological-Infectious Hazardous Waste Classification and Handling Specifications. DOF 14-09-2005. Universal Vaccination 20. Norma Oficial Mexicana NOM-031-SSA2-2009, Para la Atención de la Salud del Niño. DOF 26-09-2006. Official Mexican Standard NOM-051-SSA1-1993. Establishing the sanitary specifications for disposable sterile plastic syringes. DOF 16-01-1995.(23)

Opportunity for missed immunizations (OPPV) are defined as all circumstances in which a child under five years of age or a woman of childbearing age, even though they are eligible and in need of vaccination, are not vaccinated when they visit a health facility or service. (37,38)

BCG

Bacillus Calmette and Guérin, better known by its acronym BCG, is a vaccine against tuberculosis.is the vaccine against tuberculosis. This vaccine is prepared from an attenuated strain of *Mycobacterium bovis* which has lost its virulence in artificial cultures, maintaining its antigenic power. The vaccine is presented in an amber ampoule or vial containing 1 mg of lyophilized vaccine (10 doses) together with 1 ml of isotonic saline solution for injection (diluent) in the same physical presentation.

It is applied in newborns, or as soon as possible after birth, in a single dose of 0.1 ml. In this case it is applied intradermally in the deltoid of the right arm (upper region of the deltoid muscle) and without previous tuberculin test. It is indicated in endemic countries, in all children in the neonatal period; it can also be applied later, as long as it is before the first year of life.

Contraindications in the newborn are: premature infants with birth weight less than 2000 g, advanced malnutrition, skin conditions at the site of application, leukemia or lymphoma patients, patients with immunosuppressive treatment (corticosteroids, antimetabolites, alkylating agent, radiation), patients with clinical picture of AIDS. Asymptomatic HIV infection is not a contraindication.

The protective effect of the vaccine can be affected by many different factors such as: methods and sites of vaccine application, environment and characteristics of the population or different BCG preparation. Therefore, the range of efficacy, according to studies, varies between 0% and 80%. In children, protective efficacy rates range from 52% to 100% for tuberculous meningitis and miliary tuberculosis, and from 2% to 80% for pulmonary tuberculosis. After intradermal injection, the bacillus multiplies at the site of inoculation, and through the lymphatics reaches the regional lymph nodes, disseminating hematogenously, creating small foci in different organs.(39-42)

Anti-Hepatitis B

Hepatitis B vaccine is a vaccine developed for the prevention of hepatitis B infection. The vaccine contains one of the envelope proteins of the hepatitis B virus, the hepatitis B surface antigen. After the course of three injected doses, it is expected that the immune system will have created antibodies against HBsAg and have become established in the blood circulation.

The hepatitis B virus can survive outside the body for at least seven days, during which time it can still cause infection if it enters the body of a person not protected by the vaccine. The hepatitis B virus is transmitted through direct contact with infected body fluids, usually through a needle stick or sexual contact, not through contaminated food or water, or casual contact in the workplace.

The average incubation period for hepatitis B is 75 days, but can range from 30 to 180 days. The virus, which can be detected 30 to 60 days after infection, persists for a variable period of time. Following the primary course of three doses, a blood test is performed at an interval of 1-4 months to establish whether an adequate immune response, defined as anti-HBsAg antibody levels above 100 mIU/ml, has set in.

A complete response of this type is expected in approximately 85-90% of vaccinees. An antibody concentration between 10 and 100 mIU/ml is considered an inadequate response and it is recommended that such individuals receive an additional dose without requiring additional blood tests. Those who do not respond to the vaccine, i.e., whose blood antibody levels are less than 10 mIU/ml, should be tested to rule out present or past hepatitis B infection and should repeat the course of immunization against the virus, as well as a reassessment of their antibody levels 1 to 4 months after the second course of the vaccine. (43-47)

Anti-Rotavirus

Rotaviruses are the most common cause of diarrhea associated with vomiting and/or fever in children. Rotavirus infection primarily affects children under 5 years of age, with the child under 3 years of age being the individual most at risk of experiencing symptomatic infection, especially before 24 months of age. A child may have 5 episodes of rotavirus infection before the age of 5 years, but the first episode is often associated with greater severity.

A primary infection may present with profuse vomiting, and/or watery diarrhea with or without mucus, and/or fever that may reach 40° C or higher, with dehydration being the most significant risk. Primary infection can cause, however, a spectrum of illness ranging from mild, moderate or severe asymptomatic infection (viral shedding without symptoms), and even, as more recently described, course with viremia, which seems to occur frequently in rotavirus infections.

Reinfections tend to be mostly milder or asymptomatic, manifesting by viral shedding in the absence of symptoms. (43-47) The development of anti-rotavirus vaccines has been a long and tortuous road marked by the abrupt fall of Rotashield in 1999 due to its association with intussusception. After six years of intense research, the world is celebrating the licensure of two new vaccines that, although different in formulation and delivery, have been shown to be safe and not associated with intussusception in large Phase III studies enrolling more than 60,000 children. These two vaccines, Rotarix® from Glaxo SmithKline Biologicals and Rotateq® from Merck Sharp & Dohme are highly effective against severe diarrhea caused by rotaviruses of the most prevalent serotypes in the world. The introduction of these vaccines, sooner rather than later, especially in the poorest countries of the world, will require a joint effort by governments, manufacturing laboratories, international and non-governmental organizations and charitable foundations. (48-51)

Anti-Influenza

It is a trivalent viral vaccine prepared from influenza viruses propagated in chick embryos. It contains purified antigenic fractions (subvirions) of inactivated influenza viruses of the strains most likely to cause influenza infections in the winter following its application and which vary from year to year. Route of administration intramuscular, older than 36 months, one dose of 0.5 ml.

Antibodies increase two weeks after administration in children and three weeks in adults. When vaccine virus strains match circulating viruses, the vaccine protects 45 to 90% of healthy children and 90% of healthy adults under 65 years of age. In the elderly, it prevents illness in 30 to 70%, hospitalization in 50 to 60% and prevents influenza-associated deaths in 80% of cases. The protective effect against influenza lasts for one year. Indications Active immunization against influenza virus subtypes A and B, contained in the vaccine, in persons older than six months of age and in those who are at high risk for the disease.

Contraindicated in cases of hypersensitivity to egg proteins or to any component of the vaccine, history of Guillain-Barré syndrome, chronic cardiovascular disease, severe asthma, immunodeficiency associated disease. Do not administer during active disease of the nervous system. It is recommended to vaccinate in the last quarter of the year (October-December). All children aged six to 35 months; children aged three to nine years in high-risk conditions should be vaccinated; not recommended in pregnant women, unless the benefit outweighs the risk.

Adverse reactions frequent: local at the injection site, general malaise, headache, muscle pain rare, fever, convulsions due to fever ; rare: anaphylaxis, Guillain-Barre syndrome, asthma exacerbation , warnings for the patient the vaccine should not be administered if there has been a previous allergic reaction to influenza vaccine or in case of egg allergy. The vaccine should not be administered if pregnant. The vaccine should not be administered if the patient is being treated with drugs that suppress immunity, such as corticosteroids, unless the physician considers it a higher risk not to be vaccinated . (52-55)

Pneumococcal Conjugate Antibody

Pneumococcal disease is caused by bacteria that can spread from one person to another through close contact. It can cause ear infections and also more serious infections in the lungs (pneumonia); blood (bacteremia); the lining of the brain and spinal cord (meningitis).

Pneumococcal meningitis can cause deafness and brain damage, and kills about 1 in 10 children who get it. Everyone can get pneumococcal disease, but children under 2 years of age are at highest risk. Since the vaccine has been available, severe childhood pneumococcal disease has been reduced by 88%. Treatment of pneumococcal infections with penicillin and other drugs is not as effective as it used to be because some strains of the disease have become resistant to these drugs.

PCV13

The pneumococcal conjugate vaccine (called PCV13) provides protection against 13 types of pneumococcal bacteria. It is routinely administered to children aged 2, 4 and 6 months, and 12 to 15 months. It is also recommended for children and adults aged 2 to 64 years with certain health conditions and for all adults over 65 years of age. Persons who have had a life-threatening allergic reaction to a dose of this vaccine, to a previous pneumococcal vaccine called PCV7 (or Prevnar), or to any vaccine containing diphtheria toxoid (e.g., DTaP) should not receive PCV13. Anyone with a severe allergic reaction to any component of PCV13 should not receive this vaccine.

Reactions after vaccination: with any medication, including vaccines, reactions are likely to occur, usually mild and go away on their own, but serious reactions are also possible, with reported problems with PCV13 varying by age and dose in the series. The most frequent problems reported in children were: drowsiness after injection, a temporary loss of appetite or presented redness or tenderness at the injection site, swelling at the injection site, moderate fever (39 °C), irritability. (56)

Triple Viral

The MMR vaccine or MMR vaccine (also known as MMR and SRP) is a mixture of three attenuated viral components, administered by injection for immunization against measles (measles vaccine), mumps (mumps vaccine) and rubella (rubella vaccine). It is usually given to children at about one year of age, with a booster before the start of preschool at four to five years of age. It is a vaccine routinely used around the world.

The MMR vaccine against measles, mumps and rubella is administered subcutaneously before the age of two years, usually at one year of age, a second booster dose is necessary to achieve satisfactory levels of immunity and interrupt virus transmission, the booster can be given at one month or after one or more years, according to the individual regulations of each country.(1)

The route of administration is subcutaneous, the disinfectant used on the skin must be allowed to evaporate, since inactivation of the attenuated viruses of the vaccine may occur, it cannot be administered intradermally because immunogenicity is reduced, caution with intravenous administration, since an anaphylactic reaction may occur.

Contraindications in pregnant women should not receive the vaccine, likewise pregnancy should be avoided in the three months following vaccination, anaphylaxis to egg proteins, there are contraindications derived from each of the components, such as assessing the risk/benefit ratio in its administration to immunodeficient, the vaccine interacts with gamma globulins and blood products (even administered three months before, they can inactivate the vaccine), immunosuppressive therapy can affect immunization. It can be administered simultaneously with any of the vaccines of the immunization schedule DTP, Hib, hepatitis B, OPV, and also with the vaccine against hepatitis C.and also with varicella (chickenpox) vaccine. (57)

Adverse reactions are local and general reactions of injectable vaccines, such as fever of variable intensity (between 4 and 12 days after vaccination) due to measles virus replication, transient arthralgias may appear in young people due to rubella virus, parotid swelling caused by mumps virus, attenuated virus vaccines cause some temporary depression of general immunity, it is always necessary to assess the risk/benefit ratio. (1)

Preservation processes such as hyperattenuation of viruses make them very labile to light and heat; and the lyophilized vial should be stored between +2 °C and + 8 °C and it is recommended not to freeze. and + 8 °C and it is recommended not to freeze. (26,58)

Pentavalent Acellular

The pentavalent vaccine DPT-HB+Hib is a combined vaccine against diphtheria, pertussis, tetanus, hepatitis B and Haemophilus influenzae type B. It is obtained by mixing the tetravalent vaccine (combined vaccine against diphtheria, tetanus, pertussis and hepatitis B) with the vaccine against Haemophilus influenzae type b moments before its administration.

The tetravalent vaccine is a combination of diphtheria and tetanus anatoxins, hepatitis B virus surface antigen (recombinant) and Bordetella pertussis antigens, adsorbed in aluminum hydroxide and dissolved in an isotonic solution of sodium chloride and phosphate. (58)

The vaccine against Haemophilus influenzae type b is a conjugate vaccine composed of synthetic oligosaccharides representing fragments of the natural capsular polysaccharide. The oligosaccharides are conjugated to the carrier protein tetanus anatoxin. Intramuscular route, the usual route of application is intramuscular according to the age of the child. Immunity according to clinical trials, high titers of protective antibodies were achieved for the five antigenic components that make up the vaccine. A high level of hyperresponse was obtained (> 100 IU/ml) for the Hepatitis B antigen and long-term seroprotection (≥1 µg/ml) against Hib antigen. Post-vaccination effects Based on safety evaluation and population studies, the reactogenicity profile is similar to that reported for vaccines of this type.

Systemic adverse events predominated: fever, febrile fever and local reactions, occurring mainly after the first dose, and in the first 24 hours after the administration of each dose. The adverse effects observed were of short duration, and disappear without treatment. (6-8,59)

Triple Bacterial: (DPT)

It is a mixture of three vaccines that immunize against diphtheria, *Bordetella pertussis* (whooping cough/pertussis) and tetanus. Children should receive five doses of DPT: at 2 months of age, then at 4 months, at 11 months (these three DPTs are included in the vaccine called pentavalent), at 18 months and at 4-6 years DPT is a vaccine against diphtheria, pertussis and tetanus, so it is used in active immunization against these three diseases. The dose is 0.5 ml with 30 Lf (flocculation units) of diphtheria toxoid, 25 Lf of tetanus toxoid and the corresponding 10 to 10 x 10^9 cells of Bordetella pertussis in the case of whole cell vaccine, adsorbed in aluminum salts gel. It is administered by deep intramuscular route. (55)

Route of administration is intramuscular. It should be applied in the middle third of the external anterolateral face of the right thigh in children under 18 months of age. For older than 18 months of age and depending on their muscle mass, apply in the deltoid region of the right arm. Dose: 0.5 ml of reconstituted vaccine, reactions to DPT vaccine are provoked by the pertussis component. Moderate reactions to DPT vaccine may occur in 0.1 to 1% of vaccinated patients, including crying for more than three hours and fever up to 40 °C. Severe reactions following DPT vaccination are very rare and include severe allergic reactions, seizures, decreased consciousness and even death. These severe neurological events occur in about 1 in 140'000 doses of DPT. (7,8)

COVID-19 Vaccine

The COVID-19 vaccine In June, the FDA licensed and CDC recommended the Moderna and Pfizer-BioNTech vaccines for the 6-month to 5-year age group, expanding eligibility for vaccination to most Americans.

Pfizer-BioNTech

- Age range: 6 months to 4 years.
- Number of vaccinations: three (with an interval of three weeks between the first and second vaccination, and an interval of at least eight weeks between the second and third vaccination).
- Dose: three micrograms in each vaccine (1/10 of the adult dose).

Modern

- Age range: 6 months to 5 years.
- Number of vaccinations: two (with an interval of four weeks between the first and second vaccination).
- Dose: 25 micrograms in each vaccine (1/4 of the adult dose). (60,61)

Novavax COVID-19 vaccine is available under emergency use authorization (EUAThe vaccine is licensed for emergency use to prevent COVID-19 in persons 12 years of age and older. The vaccine is licensed for emergency use to provide: A two-dose core vaccination schedule for persons 12 years of age and older.

A first booster dose for the following individuals at least 6 months after completion of the primary vaccination schedule with a licensed or approved COVID-19 vaccine: Individuals 18 years of age and older for whom an FDA-licensed bivalent mRNA COVID-19 booster vaccine is not accessible or clinically appropriate.

licensed by the FDA is not accessible or clinically appropriate. They also choose to receive Novavax COVID-19 vaccine with adjuvant because they would not otherwise receive a booster dose of a COVID-19 vaccine.

With adjuvant contains the SARS-CoV-2 spicule protein and Matrix-M adjuvant. Adjuvants are incorporated into some vaccines to enhance the immune response of the vaccinated individual. The spicule protein in this vaccine is produced in insect cells; the Matrix-M adjuvant contains saponin extracts from the bark of the Soapbark tree that is native to Chile.(61)

The CanSino vaccine can be offered to persons who have passed COVID-19, but those persons may wish to delay vaccination until 3 months after infection. The SAGE-recommended schedule for Ad5-nCoV vaccine is a single dose (0.5 ml) administered intramuscularly in the deltoid muscle.

The U.S. Food and Drug Administration (FDA) approved Pfizer-BioNTech's COVID-19 vaccine, now called Comirnaty, to prevent COVID-19 in people 12 years of age and older. The vaccine is licensed for emergency use in children aged 6 months to 11 years. The FDA also approved Moderna's vaccine, now called Spikevax, to prevent COVID-19 in people 18 years and older. (60)

FDA authorized emergency use of Moderna's COVID-19 vaccines for children 6 months through 17 years of age. FDA authorized emergency use of Johnson & Johnson's Janssen COVID-19 vaccine for certain persons 18 years of age and older. The FDA also licensed emergency use of Novavax's COVID-19 adjuvanted vaccine for persons 12 years of age and older. (60,61)

1.6.3 Vaccination schedule at Mexico

In the following paragraphs we will discuss the different vaccines given to children under 5 years of age in the United Mexican States.

Table 1
Different types of vaccines.

Biological	Indication	Dosage and route of administration	Contraindications
BCG	Tuberculosis (miliary and meningeal)	Single dose of 0.1 ml Intradermal route Right arm deltoid region	Febrile conditions Patients with congenital or acquired immunodeficiencies Do not apply during pregnancy.
Hepatitis B	Acute and chronic hepatitis, liver failure and cirrhosis and hepatocellular carcinoma; especially for newborns born to AgsHb-positive mothers.	Children: 5 or 10 mg in 0.5 ml Adolescents: 20 mg in 1 ml. Intramuscular route, Children under 18 months apply on the external anterolateral side of the left thigh, Older than 18 months, in the deltoid region of the right arm.	Persons with a history of hypersensitivity to one or more components of the vaccine. Moderate or severe illness with or without fever.
Acellular Pentavalent Vaccine DPaT+VIP+ Hib	Active immunization against diphtheria, pertussis, tetanus, polio and invasive Haemophilus influenza type b infections.	Dosage: 0.5 ml reconstituted Intramuscular use Apply in the middle third of the external anterolateral face of the right thigh in children under 18 months of age. Older than 18 months of age and depending on their muscle mass, apply in the deltoid region of the right arm.	Anaphylactic reaction following vaccine administration, allergy to neomycin, streptomycin or polymyxin B, fever of 38.5 °C.
DPT: Whole cell pertussis vaccine with diphtheria and tetanus toxoids.	Active booster immunization against diphtheria, pertussis and tetanus.	Dosage: 0.5 ml Intramuscular **route** Apply to the deltoid region of the left arm.	Do not apply to children over 6 years 11 months of age. Immediate anaphylactic reaction. Encephalopathy (cause not identified). Progressive neurological disease, seizures.
Vaccine Antirrotavirus	Prevention of gastroenteritis caused by rotavirus	Dosage: 1.5 or 2 ml Oral route	Hypersensitivity to previous administration Persons with uncorrected congenital malformations of the gastrointestinal tract.
Vaccine Pneumococcal conjugate.	Active immunization against invasive pneumococcal infections caused by Streptococcus pneumoniae of the serotypes included in the vaccine.	Dosage is 0.5 ml Intramuscular route Under 18 months in the middle third of the anterolateral external aspect of the right thigh.	Hypersensitivity to the active ingredients or any of the excipients of the formula, acute febrile conditions (above 38.5 °C).

Biological	Indication	Dosage and route of administration	Contraindications
		Older than 18 months apply in the deltoid region of the arm.	
Vaccine Anti-influenza of whole, fractionated and subunit viruses (seasonal use).	Active immunization against influenza virus types A and B infection	Children from 6 to 35 months of age will receive two doses of 0.25 ml. For subsequent annual vaccination they will receive a dose of 0.25 ml through an intramuscular route of administration, for the population from 6 to 18 months of age.	Hypersensitivity to any of the components, infants younger than 6 months, history of Guillain Barré syndrome, acute febrile illness, with fever greater than 38.5 °C, moderate or severe acute illness with or without fever.
Vaccine MMR, Anti Measles, Anti-Rubella and Anti-Mumps (SRP).	Active immunization against measles, rubella and mumps.	Dosage is 0.5 ml Subcutaneous route Apply to the upper outer triceps area of the left arm.	People with immunodeficiencies acute febrile history of anaphylactic reaction to egg proteins or other components of the formula. People who have been transfused or who have received immunoglobulin should wait three to eleven months to be vaccinated.
Sabin type trivalent oral polio vaccine (OPV).	Active immunization against poliomyelitis.	Dosage of 0.1 ml, equivalent to two drops. Oral route	People with immunodeficiencies. Acute febrile illnesses Allergic reactions to previous doses.
Double viral vaccine, Anti-measles and Anti-rubella (SR).	Active immunization against measles and rubella.	Dosage of 0.5 ml Subcutaneous route, Apply to the upper outer triceps area of the left arm.	Persons with immunodeficiencies, except HIV infection in asymptomatic state; acute febrile conditions, persons suffering from leukemia (except if in remission and have not received chemotherapy in the last three months), anaphylactic reaction to egg protein Transfused or immunoglobulin recipients should wait 3 to 11 months to be vaccinated.
Acellular Pertussis vaccine with diphtheria and	Active immunization against diphtheria, pertussis and tetanus.	Dosage of 0.5 ml Intramuscular route. Under 18 months of age in the middle third of the	Hypersensitivity to the formulation, In such cases, DT vaccine should be administered for the

Biological	Indication	Dosage and route of administration	Contraindications
tetanus toxoids (DPaT)		external anterolateral aspect of the thigh; over 18 months of age and, depending on muscle mass; apply in the deltoid region.	remaining doses in the vaccination schedule to ensure protection against diphtheria and tetanus.

Source: Secretariat of Health 2021

Table 2 below specifies the vaccines corresponding to age, the National Immunization Schedule 2022 for children under 10 years of age.

Table 2
National Vaccination Schedule

Age	Vaccines			
Birth	BCG	Hepatitis B		
2 months	Pentavalent Acellular	Hepatitis B	Rotavirus	Pneumococcal conjugate
4 months	Pentavalent Acellular		Rotavirus	Pneumococcal conjugate
6 months	Pentavalent Acellular	Hepatitis B	Rotavirus	Influenza
7 months	Influenza second dose			
12 months	SRP			Pneumococcal conjugate
18 months	Pentavalent Acellular			
24 months	Influenza annual booster			
36 months	Influenza annual booster			
48 months	DPT (Booster)			Influenza annual booster
59 months	Annual influenza booster VOP (Oral Polio) from 6 to 59 months in 1st and 2nd National Health Week.			
72 months	SRP (reinforcement)			
6 to 11 years	COVID-19 (2 doses) 3-8 weeks after 1st dose Bivalent booster dose at least 2 months after the last dose(s)			
11 years old or 5th year of primary school	HPV (Human Papilloma Virus)			

Source: Secretariat of Health 202 1

1.5.4 Factors involved in the mother's attendance or non-attendance at immunizations

Sociodemographic and cultural factors.

Social factors. Set of norms, laws, principles that determine or influence the conduct or behavior of individuals in a society. Said of those qualities that serve to distinguish someone or something from their peers. It includes the following: Occupation and marital status. (20)

Occupation. Employment or activity, whether paid or unpaid, performed by a person. Classifying them as: Housewife. Persons who, without exercising any economic activity, dedicate themselves to taking care of their own homes. These people dedicate themselves solely and exclusively to domestic chores or household chores, are not looking for work, are not pensioned or retired, do not receive income, and do not attend basic education school; according to a private worker.

Private sector employees are those who are located in places that are not government agencies. These may include both individual business owners and other forms of company organizations, such as corporations or limited partnerships. Public Worker. Any natural person who renders personal services in the social process of work under the dependence of a government institution. Student. A person who is dedicated solely and exclusively to study. (21)

Civil status. It is the quality of an individual, in that it enables or disables him to exercise certain rights or to contract certain civil obligations; in such a way that according to this concept the civil status is the one that imprints the character to the individual, emanating from the fact that constitutes it, conferring him a set of rights and obligations proper to his person, as a quality of this, while the capacity is the aptitude or faculty to exercise by himself his rights. (18,22,23)

There are different types of marital status that vary according to the type of relationships a person has with others. Among the most common are. Single: Those who are not legally committed to others. Married: A person who has contracted a civil or ecclesiastical marriage.

Union libre: This is the term used for people who have been living together for more than 2 years. Divorced: A person who has broken the legal bond with his or her partner. Widowed: A person who has no partner as a result of the death of a spouse. (21)

Demographic factors.

Age. It is the time elapsed between the birth of an individual and the present moment, it is measured in days, months or years and is determined by different stages. Among them: adolescent (between 11 and 19 years), young (between 20 and 30 years) and adult (between 31 and 50 years), older adults (over 51 years). (24)

Number of children. Refers to the total number of children born alive that the mother has had up to the moment she registers her last child. Level of education. According to J. Brunner, the level of education is the level of systematic schooling and constitutes the last grade completed and approved by the person. It is classified as follows: Without instruction*:* when the person knows how to read and write, but has not completed any type of studies. Primary: the person has completed or incomplete primary education. Secondary: the person attained complete or incomplete secondary education. Higher or professional: the person has attained a higher university and/or technical education, complete or incomplete. (24)

Knowledge: the dictionary of the Royal Spanish Academy defines knowledge as the action of knowing; to know is to acquire the notion of things through understanding. It is a relationship established between the knowing subject and the known object. Knowledge has an individual and social character; it can be: personal, group and organizational, since each person interprets the information he/she perceives on the basis of his/her past experience, influenced by the groups to which he/she belonged and belongs. They are also influenced by the acceptance patterns that form the culture of their organization and the social values in which they have spent their lives. (10)

The information they receive about immunizations: many families lack reliable information about immunizations and immunization services; they often do not know that if they miss a scheduled immunization appointment they can still be immunized; they should just go as soon as possible to get vaccinated. (20)

The following are common misconceptions: children are protected against vaccine-preventable diseases by a religious or supernatural being watching over them, children are fully protected because they have already received some immunizations, sick children cannot be vaccinated, immunizations often cause sterilization, illness or dangerous adverse effects, parents do not know that the child can be vaccinated at any health unit in the country for follow-up. (4,25)

Parents believe that they have to pay for consultations in order to vaccinate their children; health services would come to their home or community if vaccination were really important, as they do during campaigns. Local health workers have a particularly important role in improving people's level of awareness and providing information to beneficiary populations; information should be given in general terms: vaccines and diseases they prevent, vaccination schedule, importance, receiving it on time; all this in appropriate language; it is an effective measure. (3)

Pediatric factors

A very important aspect related to the safety of vaccines are the precautions and contraindications of each vaccine in order to avoid situations that may put the patient at risk.

Contraindications: A condition of the individual that significantly increases the risk of suffering a serious adverse effect if given a particular vaccine, most contraindications are temporary and once that situation has passed the patient can be vaccinated.(24)

Temporary contraindications: Temporary contraindications allow the administration of a vaccine once they are resolved. Any moderate or severe disease (asthmatic crisis, decompensated cardiopathy, acute diarrhea), with or without fever, is a temporary contraindication for the administration of vaccines, except in situations of very high epidemic risk. Once the situation has disappeared, vaccines can be administered. (19)

The age of administration may be considered a contraindication. It is not advisable to administer the MMR vaccine before 12 months of age because it may interfere with maternal antibodies and not produce a complete immune response, although in epidemic situations it can be administered from 6 months of age, although two doses should be administered after 12 months of age. Similarly, the hepatitis A vaccine is administered from 12 months of age, the influenza vaccine from 6 months of age and the standard diphtheria and pertussis (D and P) antigen load components can only be administered up to 7 years of age.(24)

Precautions: these are situations in which the administration of a vaccine entails an increased risk of presenting an adverse effect or that the immune response to the vaccine may be insufficient and not allow adequate protection to be obtained.

Some situations considered precautions are: Hypotonia-hypo responsive picture (shock-like picture) or fever greater than 40.5 °C or persistent crying picture of 3 or more hours within 48 hours, or seizures within 72 hours after administration of a dose of any vaccine with pertussis component. Progressive neurological disorder, including infantile spasms, uncontrolled epilepsy, and progressive encephalopathy. In these cases it is recommended to delay vaccination until stabilization of the process. (3,15,16,26,27)

Patients with chronic diseases and/or immunosuppression: the response to vaccination may be suboptimal in some of these patients, so vaccines should be administered taking this fact into account. It has been previously mentioned that in case of immunosuppression attenuated vaccines are contraindicated in most situations.

The administration of biological products (immunoglobulins or blood) prior to the administration of MMR or varicella vaccine. An exception to anaphylaxis as a contraindication are children with anaphylactic allergy to eggs, since they can receive the MMR vaccine at the health center, because it has practically no egg proteins, although they must wait 15-30 minutes in the waiting room as with all vaccines. (27-30)

1.5.5 The Caregiver

Caregivers care for children and infants whose parents or guardians go to work. In addition to providing basic care with practical responsibilities such as washing, dressing, and feeding, they foster children's social and educational development and provide a safe and stimulating environment for learning and playing.(20)

Child caregivers provide a safe and stimulating environment in which children can play, learn and develop new skills. They encourage children to participate in activities such as drawing or painting, reading stories and playing games. Childminders are usually licensed to care for up to six children under the age of eight. Only three of them can be under the age of five. It is important that child caregivers establish a good relationship with parents. (24)

Among these factors it is important for caregivers to link preventive care measures in their children, mainly in prevention to the use of vaccines, both parties are likely to discuss various issues such as making sure the child is happy and receives stimulation, agreeing on what kind of behavior is acceptable, planning the child's diet (e.g., if the child has any allergies), etc. In these cases, caregivers plan the use of books, toys and activities to meet the child's physical and emotional needs.

Some characteristics of caregivers are taking initiative and making decisions, staying calm under pressure and in emergency situations, showing understanding and encouragement, putting up with noise and constant demands for attention, building friendly and open relationships with children and parents, showing parents that you are trustworthy and responsible. It is useful to have knowledge of first aid, hygiene and nutrition, and it is very important to pay attention to safety. (12,31)

The child from 3 to 5 years of age, development and growth

It is a period of great enrichment in the interrelation. The child is schooled in the basic infant level school commonly called "preschool"; which implies an expansion and learning of respect for social and coexistence rules; in the motor aspects, the career becomes stable and the maturity of motor skills implies the ability to play games that require stability and balance (bicycle, ball), as well as games of social exchange with other children in their environment. (20)

The vocabulary will increase to about two thousand words; the increase in fluency, increase in vocabulary and ability to elaborate sentences of increasing number of words. Feeding varies in quantity, with days of apparent lack of appetite and others of normal intake. Therefore, the most useful thing, to avoid situations of concern and worry in parents, is to consider the average weekly intake, which is more stable, instead of measuring the specific intake of each day. (24)

Moral thinking emerges with the perception of what is right and wrong, as well as the perception of empathy towards the difficulties of others. The child begins to be aware and to adopt sympathetic attitudes towards the reality that there are not only his or her own desires and difficulties, but also those of the people around him or her.(32)

The interrelationship within the family acquires great importance: the rules to be respected, which must be clear; the sense of punishment defined as the displeasure that can produce in parents the non-acceptance of family rules or the attempt to impose childish whims; and, above all, the parents as a model constitute the most important pillar of emotional development in this period.· (12-14,33-35)

1.7 Frame of reference

An exhaustive search was carried out for research studies that show the results of the variables included in this project related to the vaccination of children from three to six years of age:

Palacios Ríos & et al 2018 in their article compliance with the national vaccination schedule in pediatric patients attending an outpatient clinic in a tertiary hospital in their cross-sectional, descriptive study in patients under 12 years of age concludes that the main reasons for non-compliance with the schedules were: hospitalization, medical indication for non-vaccination and lack of supply at the vaccination center. In adolescent girls, the human papillomavirus (HPV) vaccine has a 66% compliance rate in the first year of life.) has a compliance rate of 66% in the first two doses and only 33% in the third. (32)

Caldeóon Alarcón, Ccaccya Serna, Ccente Pérez 2021 in their research work on the relationship between sociocultural factors and compliance with the National Vaccination Scheme in children under 5 years of age attending the Health Center, Los Olivos, Lima 2021, type of non-experimental cross-sectional research, descriptive method and correlational design concludes that the variable sociocultural factors is directly and positively related to the variable compliance with the national vaccination scheme, according to Spearman's correlation of 0.673 (24)

Vallejo Carrasco 2018, in his degree thesis, factors associated with non-compliance with the vaccination schedule in children aged 0 to 5 years belonging to a health sub-center in the city of Guayaquil, the research conducted is descriptive with a prospective approach, quantitative method and cross-sectional design. The population was 50 children and their caregivers, and the factor that caused the greatest non-compliance with the vaccination schedule was time (40%) and the complication that occurred was gastroenteritis (12%). (20)

Yimam Ali, Fantahun Ayenew, Lake Ayenew, Haileab Fekadu 2020 mention poor utilization of maternal health services associated with incomplete vaccination among children aged 12-23 months in Ethiopia, Human Vaccines & Immunotherapeutics, A community based cross-sectional study was conducted in Kutaber district from August to September 2017. A total of 480 participants were selected using stratified multi-stage multi-stage sampling technique, concluded that mother/caregiver educational level, vaccination depends on mother, antenatal follow-ups, place of delivery and living near health facilities were significantly associated with incomplete vaccination. (63)

Isidro Ríos, Gutiérrez Aguado 2021, the prenatal factors associated with noncompliance with the basic vaccination schedule in children under 5 years of age. In their observational, retrospective, analytical and cross-sectional study, they concluded that the prenatal risk factors associated with noncompliance with the basic vaccination schedule in children under 5 years of age were maternal age, the number of inadequate prenatal check-ups and the pregnant woman not having received the tetanus vaccine. (64)

De Loera Díaz & et al 2021 associated the reasons for non-compliance with the basic vaccination schedule in a rural community of Aguascalientes, a qualitative, cross-sectional study through a structured interview, concluded that the reasons expressed by the mothers were diverse and many of these were referred to in previous studies, which stands out in this research and the main reason identified was disinterest in compliance. Non-compliance with the basic vaccination schedule is a multifactorial phenomenon in which health education is an indispensable issue for its resolution; being a rural community, its population becomes more vulnerable, so it is necessary to intervene in the identified reasons. (21)

Chapter 2: Methodology

The following chapter describes the design, population, instrument and procedures and how the human rights of research participants are to be protected.

2.1 Study design

This research work is a quantitative-descriptive cross-sectional design, because it is based on the deductive method in which a problem is posed based on a theoretical framework.

2.2 Population

For the development of the project, we worked with all the mothers of the kindergarten who attended during April 2023. The population was made up of kindergarten students, the sample was a total of 26 mothers who have children from 3 to 5 years old attending the "José Vasconcelos" kindergarten, the non-probabilistic sampling by disposition of the sample.

2.3 Selection criteria

Inclusion criteria

- Mothers/parents/caregivers of children 3 to 5 years old.
- They must have a vaccination card.
- Have their children attend the José Vasconcelos kindergarten.
- That they agree to participate in the survey.
- Fathers and mothers of families.
- Verbal ability to answer the questionnaire.

Exclusion criteria

- Mothers/parents/caregivers who do not have an immunization record.
- Mothers/parents/caregivers who are physically unable to speak or are unconscious.

2.4 Space and time limits

Space:
The research was conducted in a basic education school in the community of San Juan Tizahuapan, Epazoyucan, Hidalgo.

Time:
The study was conducted in children under 5 years of age, during the month of April 2023.

2.5 Evaluation instrument

Through the systematic collection of information from the questionnaire: Sociocultural Factors and their Relationship to Compliance with the National Vaccination Schedule in Children Under 5 years of age with the acronym CEIFSRCENVNMA (2023) by the author Algedones Sotelo M. E. (2018), which has a 95% reliability, validated by Crombach's Alpha 0.87 for the variables sociocultural factors and compliance with the national vaccination schedule; this consists of 38 items which was divided into: social factors with 14 items, cultural factors with 9 items, compliance with the vaccination booklet with 7 items and mother's self-discipline with 8 items, with the options A.-always, B.-sometimes, C.-very rarely, D.-never.

2.6 Data collection procedure

1. The kindergarten was selected as the center of the research project, the research protocol was presented to the directors of the kindergarten and the director was informed of the benefits of developing the project by means of a letter (annex D and E) specifying why, for what purpose and for what purposes the research would be carried out.

2. On the agreed-upon day, the mothers were informed by the director that they would bring their vaccination cards with them to collate the information. In the morning, the mothers or guardians of the children were summoned to the multipurpose room of the preschool, where they were explained how to fill out the data form (Appendix C).

3. The informed and consensual consent form was read, in which the confidentiality of the information was guaranteed (Annex B). It was

explained in detail that their participation was voluntary and that the data obtained would be used for teaching purposes, and any doubts or suggestions made by the mothers at that time were individually dispelled.

4. The instrument (Annex C) was applied to mothers/parents/caregivers of children aged 3 to 5 years with vaccination records who met the selection criteria.

5. The information was tabulated by means of the operationalization of variables (Annex A) and the preparation of statistical tables, and finally the results obtained were analyzed using SPSS, obtaining frequencies, percentages and graphs.

2.7 Ethical Considerations

The ethical aspects of this research were taken into account in accordance with the **Regulations of the General Health Law (**1987) on Research on the ethical aspects of research on human beings, contained in the second title, chapter I and chapter III.

From chapter I, according to article 13, the dignity and protection of the rights and well-being of the participants were respected; according to article 14, the research was carried out in accordance with the scientific and ethical principles that justify it. In accordance with article 17, it was considered that in this case it was a minimal risk research, since no intervention or intentional modification was made in the physiological, psychological and social variables of the participants in the study, 1 instrument was used. Informed consent was obtained from the parents and study participants, as established in article 21, and was given in writing, as indicated in article 22.

Article 100.- Research on human beings shall be developed according to the following bases.

- It should be adapted to the scientific and ethical principles that justify medical research, especially with regard to its potential contribution to the solution of health problems and the development of new fields of medical science.

- Written informed consent must be obtained from the subject on whom the research will be performed or from his/her legal representative in case of legal incapacity.

- According to the Declaration of Helsinki adopted by the 18th World Medical Assembly, which states that the main objective of health research is to generate new knowledge based on ethical principles for research on human beings.

In addition to **the** conduct of this research, the ethical aspects supported by the **Declaration of Helsinki** were taken into account, as can be seen in the following information:

Medical research is subject to ethical standards that serve to promote respect for all human beings and to protect their health and individual rights. Some research populations are vulnerable and need special protection. The particular needs of the economically and medically disadvantaged must be recognized.

Special attention should also be given to those who cannot give or refuse consent on their own, those who may give consent under duress, those who will not personally benefit from the research, and those who have research combined with medical care.

Ethical Principle Number 8.- Although the main objective of medical research is to generate new knowledge, this objective should never take precedence over the rights and interests of the research subject.

In medical research, it is the duty of the physician to protect the life, health, dignity, integrity, right to self-determination, privacy and confidentiality of personal information of research subjects. The responsibility for the protection of research subjects should always rest with a physician or other health care professional and never with the research participants, even if they have given their consent.

This project was conducted under the approach of a descriptive method so it is considered a research without risk, and was accepted by the management staff of the school of basic preschool education, based in the community of San Juan Tizahuapan, Epazoyucan, Hidalgo; with the official letter 190423 in which this study respects the privacy of the adult participants, children with an academic purpose. (Annex E).

2.8 Statistical analysis plan

The statistical package Statistical Package For The Social Sciences (SPSS) version 27 will be used for data analysis.) version 27, descriptive statistics will be used to measure frequencies, percentages, and some measures of central tendency and graphs; as well as inferential statistics for hypothesis testing by means of Pearson's correlation.

Chapter 3: Results

The results collected were expressed according to the variables established in tables and graphs representing percentages and inferential statistics, respectively.

3.1 Sociodemographic and cultural data

Table 5 showed that the age of the children's mothers ranged from 31 to 40 years, which is equivalent to 50%.

Regarding the marital status of the mother, it was found that 46.2% are married and only 3.8% are single; on the occupation of the mother it was found that 26.9% are engaged in household activities, 23.1% are private workers, 50% are public workers , the level of study of the mother was found that 57.7% studied a bachelor's degree, 23.1% finished high school.

It was identified that 100% speak Spanish, in the origin of the mother 46.2% come from the city and 42.3% from the municipality, in the way their family is composed we found that 69.2% live with their father, mother and children, 15.4% live at home with their mother and children, and 11.5% live with their father, mother, children and grandparents, 3.8% live at home with their father and children .

Regarding the place of birth of the child, we found that 84.6% were born in a hospital, 15.4% were born in a clinic , in how many children they have, we found that 73.1% have less than 3 children, and 26.9% have 3 or 4 children .

Table 3
Distribution of the sociodemographic factors of the population studied.

Frequency (%))

Age of Participant	19 or Less	1(3.8)
	20 a 30	9(34.6)
	From 31 to 40	13(50)
	Older than 41	3(11.5)
Marital Status	Single	1(3.8)
	Married	**12(46.2)**
	Free Union	9(34.6)
	Divorced	4(15.4)
Mother's Occupation	Housewife	7(26.9)
	Private Worker	6(23.1)
	Public Worker	**13(50)**
Schooling	Primary	1(3.8)
	Secondary	6(23.1)
	Bachelor's Degree	**15(57.7)**
	Postgraduate	4(15.4)
Monthly Family Income	Greater than $4900	**13(50)**
	From $2000 To $4800	11(42.3)
	Less than $2000	1(3.8)
	No Income	1(3.8)

Source: N=26; CEIFSRCENVNMA (2023).

In the following table 6, regarding the age of the youngest child we found that 88.5% of the children are between 2 and 5 years old, 7.7% of the children are between 8 and 15 months old, and only 3.8% of the children are 7 months old or younger.8% of their youngest child is 7 months old or less , the monthly family income we found that 50% receive an income greater than $4900, 42.3% receive a monthly income of $2000 to $4800, 3.8% receive less than $2000 pesos per month, and 3.8% do not receive any type of income .

On the other hand, 46.2% live in their own home, 30.8% live in a relative's home, and 23.1% live in a borrowed home .

To take their child to vaccination, what transportation do they use, 38.5% go to vaccinate their children in private transportation, 34.6% go to vaccinate their children on foot, 15.4% by bus and only 11.5% by cab , as to whether they have heard publicity regarding vaccination that their child should take to vaccination 53.8% sometimes, 46.2% always.

Table 4
Distribution of the social factors of the population studied.

Frequency (%)

Native Language	**Spanish**	**26(100)**
Mother's origin	Colony Municipality City	3(11.5) 11(42.3) **12(46.2)**
His family is composed of	Dad, Mom and Children Mom and Kids Dad and Sons Dad, Mom, Children and Grandparents	**18(62.9)** 4(15.4) 1(3.8) 3(11.5)
Child's place of birth	Clinic Hospital	4(15.4) **22(84.6)**
Number of children	Less than 3 3 o 4	**19(73.1)** 7(26.9)
Age of youngest child	7 Months or Less From 8 to 15 Months From 2 to 5 Years	1(3.8) 2(7.7) **23(88.5)**
The house you live in is	Own From a Family Member Borrowed	**12 (46.2)** 8(30.8) 6(23.1)
Type of transport used	Private Transportation On Foot Bus Cab	**10(38.5)** 9(34,6) 4(15.4) 3(11.5)
If you have heard vaccination advertising	Sometimes Always	**14(53.8)** 12(46.2)

Source: N=26; CEIFSRCENVNMA (2023).

3.2 National Immunization Schedule for schoolchildren under 5 years of age

We found in the following graph 3, that 84.6% always in their family take their children to be vaccinated, 11.5% sometimes, and 3.8% never, 61.5% do not consider that receiving several vaccines weakens the immune system, and 16.4% sometimes consider it, 80.8% take their children to be vaccinated.

Even if other people advise against it, 100% believe it is necessary to give replacement vaccines, 3.8% very rarely consider home-made medicines as a substitute for vaccines, and 100% never consider vaccines to be dangerous and harmful to health.

Graph 3

Cultural factors (customs and habits) of the population studied.

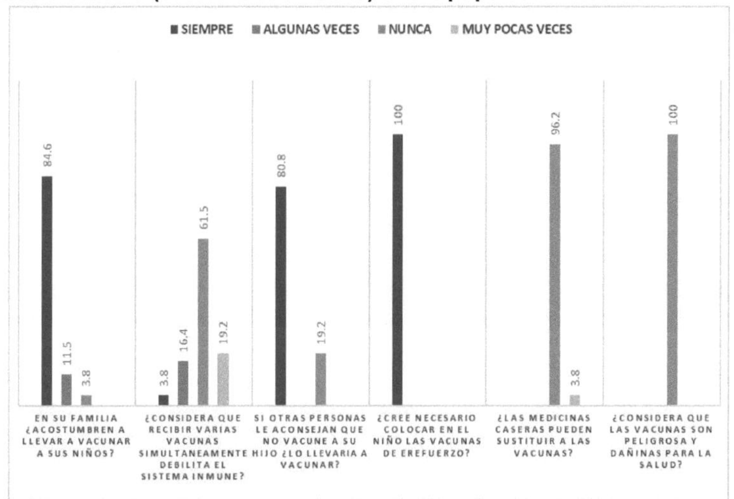

Source: N=26; CEIFSRCENVNMA (2023).

Graph 4 showed that 84.6% have so far complied with taking their child to be vaccinated on the scheduled date and 15.4% sometimes, 88.5% always feel committed to keep vaccination appointments and the same number feel committed to be informed about the benefits of vaccines, 80.8%.

On the other hand, they have time to take their children to vaccinations and 15.4% sometimes, 38.5% would sometimes take their child to a relative if they could not take them to vaccinations, and 19.2% would never take them, 96.2% would never believe that homemade medicines could substitute vaccinations, 76.9% always look for a way to find a solution if they cannot keep the vaccination appointment.

Graph 4
Compliance with the vaccination card of the population studied.

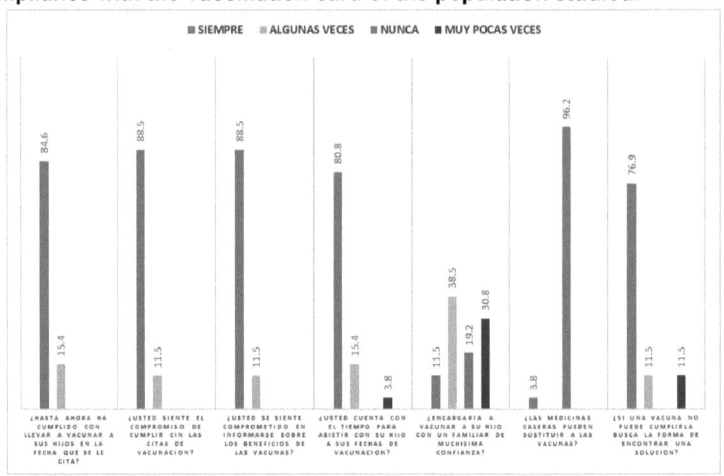

Source: N=26; CEIFSRCENVNMA (2023).

Graph 5 shows that 73.1% always attend scheduled vaccination appointments and 3.8% never attend, while 80.8% always maintain continuity in the vaccination schedule.

The population that participated in the study, 92.3% never consider vaccines to be dangerous and harmful to health, 69.2% keep track of their vaccination appointments and 16.4% never keep track, 65.4% never blame other diseases on vaccines and 3.8% always do, 57.7% never self-medicate their child and 3.8% sometimes.

Graph 5
Self-discipline of the mother of the population studied.

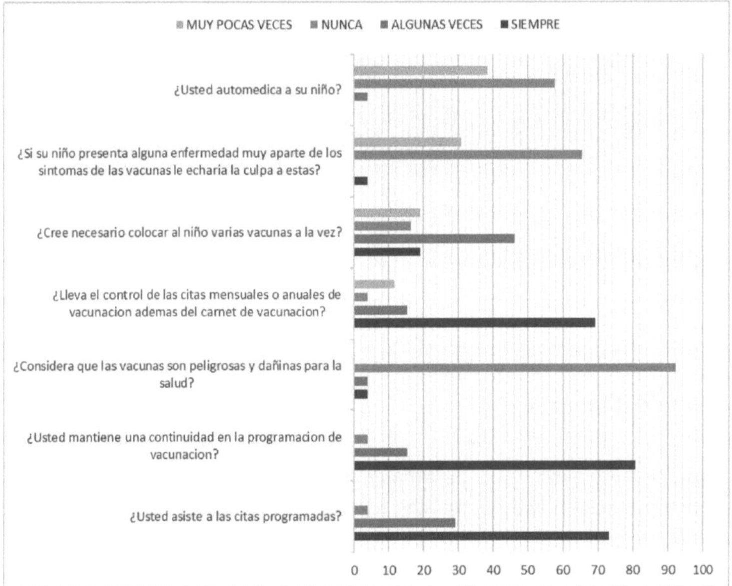

Source: N=26; CEIFSRCENVNMA (2023).

Graph 6 shows that the main reason for not keeping their vaccination appointment was not remembering the date (26.9%) and the same percentage did not keep their appointments, lack of time (23.1%), difficulty in getting there (19.2%), and 3.8% lost their vaccination card (3.8%).

Graph 6
Reason for noncompliance of the population studied.

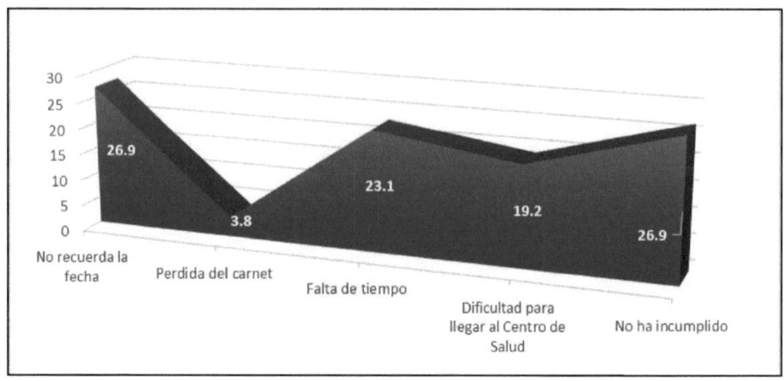

Source: N=26; CEIFSRCENVNMA (2023).

3.3 Inferential Statistics

Pearson's correlation is a parametric statistical method that measures the relationship between two quantitative variables; Pearson's correlation coefficient ranges from -1 to +1, and its value indicates the type of correlation and its strength:

- Negative correlation: A value less than 0 indicates a negative correlation.
- Positive correlation: A value greater than 0 indicates a positive correlation.
- No linear relationship: A value of 0, or close to 0, indicates that there is no linear relationship between the two variables.

To calculate Pearson's correlation coefficient, certain requirements must be met, such as:

- The measurement scale should be an interval or ratio scale.
- The variables should be distributed approximately.
- The association must be linear.
- There should be no outliers in the data.

For the test of the hypothesis that cultural factors influence vaccination schedule compliance, we found a *P* value of .005 and a significance of .001. This indicates a strong positive correlation between cultural factors and compliance with the vaccination schedule.

In Table 7 we observe that for the test of H1 where the variable, they usually take their children to be vaccinated, is included, the P value is 0.044, with a significance of 0.726, indicating a strong positive correlation.

Table 5
Cultural Factors

		Value and Description
In the event that your child misses his or her immunization appointment, you consider that:	In your family, do you usually take your children to be vaccinated?	.726 Strong positive correlation.
Do you think it is necessary to give the child booster vaccines?	In your family, do you usually take your children to be vaccinated?	.411 Weak positive correlation.
Do you consider vaccines to be dangerous and harmful to health?	In your family, do you usually take your children to be vaccinated?	.646 Mean positive correlation.
	In the event that your child misses his or her immunization appointment, you consider that	.519 Mean positive correlation.
	Can home-made medicines replace vaccines?	.483 Weak positive correlation.

Source: N=26. CEIFSRCENVNMA (2023).

Table 8 shows that for the test of H1, the variable maintains continuity in the vaccination schedule, the P value is 0.039, with a significance of 0.533 mean positive correlation.

Table 6
Mother's self-discipline

		Value and Description
Do you consider vaccines to be dangerous and harmful to health?	Do you maintain continuity in vaccination scheduling?	0.494 weak positive correlation
What is the main reason you missed your vaccination appointment?	Do you attend scheduled appointments?	0.462 weak positive correlation
	Do you keep track of monthly or annual immunization appointments in addition to the immunization record?	0.533 average positive correlation.
	Do you self-medicate your child?	0.400 weak positive correlation

Source: N=26. CEIFSRCENVNMA (2023).

With this, hypothesis H1 is tested; where "keeps track of monthly or annual vaccination appointments in addition to the vaccination card"; obtaining a correlation of 0.533 positive mean.

Chapter 4: Conclusions

4.1 Discussion

The information obtained from the results was analyzed, to later make a discussion of these results with the references obtained during the research process, thus identifying trends and discrepancies that allow making a contribution to this field of knowledge, as well as established in the objectives, allows identifying factors that influence non-compliance with the vaccination schedule in children under 5 years of age in a basic education school in the community of San Juan Tizahuapan, Epazoyucan Hidalgo.

According to the results obtained in this research, with respect to sociocultural factors related to compliance with the vaccination schedule, the age of the mother of the children oscillates in the range of 30 to 40 years with 50%. Being different from the results of Isidro Rios, Gutierrez Aguado 2021, where he found less than half are younger with the highest percentage (42%) of the surveyed mothers attending the health center are very young with less than 20 years. (64)

Calderón Alarcón, Ccaccya Serna, Ccente Pérez 2021 in their research work on the relationship between sociocultural factors and compliance with the National Vaccination Scheme in children under 5 years of age, it was found that the variable sociocultural factors is directly and positively related to the variable compliance with the national vaccination scheme, similar to the findings reported in this study where it refers to the mother's perspective on the use of vaccines: 89% believe that vaccines are necessary because they prevent or protect against serious diseases, 61.5% believe that vaccines never weaken the immune system, 100% believe that booster vaccines are necessary, and 100% believe that vaccines are never harmful. It was observed that mothers did comply with the vaccination schedule, therefore, immunopreventable diseases may be higher in their children who are not protected. (24)

De Loera Díaz & et al 2021, associated the reasons for non-compliance with the basic vaccination schedule in a rural community of Aguascalientes, a qualitative, cross-sectional study through a structured interview, concluded that the reasons expressed by the mothers were diverse and many of these referred to in previous studies, which stands out in this research and the main reason identified was disinterest in compliance. In the results found, 26.9% have not complied with the vaccination card, the same number have not remembered the date and 23.1% have not complied due to lack of time.(21)

The mother's self-discipline and cultural factors do influence compliance with the vaccination card. With this we verify what Nola Pender wrote in the Health Promotion Model, which explains how individual characteristics and experiences, as well as knowledge, affect the behavior that leads the individual to participate or not in health behaviors; situational factors such as knowledge and self-discipline do influence mothers' compliance with the vaccination schedule, thus accepting the hypothesis.

4.2 Conclusions

Through this research it is observed that mothers whose children attend a preschool basic education school in the community of San Juan Tizahuapan, Epazoyucan Hidalgo; more than half of them are informed about the scheme and importance of vaccination in children under 5 years of age. It can be seen that almost half of the mothers have not failed to comply with their children's vaccination dates; the main reason why those responsible for the children did not comply with the vaccination booklet was because they did not remember the date in more than half, lack of time in a quarter, and a tenth was influenced by the loss of the booklet.

The social factors that intervene in the decision of mothers or caregivers to comply with the complete vaccination schedule are the age of the mother and her academic preparation.

The cultural factors that intervene in the compliance or non-compliance with the complete vaccination schedule are the influence that the family exerts on the decision of the mother to have her children vaccinated and in this research we did not find any cultural factors that intervene in the decision to vaccinate her children and comply with the complete schedule.

There is a positive correlation between the self-discipline of the mother or caregiver of the child, such as attending scheduled appointments, maintaining continuity in the vaccination schedule, not self-medicating their children; it is concluded that there is an important relationship between the mother's self-discipline and compliance with the National Vaccination Schedule, which influences her participation in health promoting behavior and the adoption of a commitment to an action plan, as proven by Nola Pender in her Health Promotion Model.

In this study, significant differences were found between the personal, cultural, social and situational factors that influence mothers to comply with the vaccination schedule for their children; for example, the level of education of the mother, a quarter of those who have a bachelor's degree, do vaccinate their children. The variable of the mother's level of education does have an influence on compliance with the vaccination schedule for children under 5 years of age.

4.3 Suggestions

Through the study that was conducted, it was observed that mothers whose children attend basic education school; preschool based in the community of San Juan Tizahuapan, Epazoyucan, Hidalgo; more than half of them are informed about the scheme and importance of vaccination in children under 5 years of age. It can be seen that almost half of the mothers have not failed to comply with their children's vaccination dates; the main reason why those responsible for the children did not comply with the vaccination booklet was that they could not remember the date in more than half, lack of time in a quarter, and a tenth was due to the loss of the vaccination booklet.

Social factors that intervene in the decision of mothers or caregivers to comply with the complete vaccination schedule, such as the mother's age and educational background.

The cultural factors that intervene in the compliance or non-compliance with the complete vaccination schedule; the influence that the family exerts on the decision of the mother to have her children vaccinated was identified and in the study we did not find any cultural factor that intervened in the decision to vaccinate her children and comply with the complete vaccination schedule.

There is a positive correlation between the self-discipline of the mother or caregiver of the child, such as attending scheduled appointments, maintaining continuity in the vaccination schedule, not self-medicating their children; where it is concluded that there is an important relationship between the mother's self-discipline and compliance with the National Vaccination Schedule, influencing her participation in health promoting behavior; and the adoption of a commitment to an action plan; as shown by Nola Pender in her Model of Health Promotion.

In this study, significant differences were found between the personal, cultural, social and situational factors of the mothers; for example, the level of education of the mother is a factor that influences compliance with the vaccination schedule of children under 5 years of age.

References

1. Moreno-Pérez D, Álvarez García FJ, Arístegui Fernández J, Cilleruelo Ortega MJ, Corretger Rauet JM, García Sánchez N, et al. Vaccination calendar of the Spanish Association of Pediatrics (CAV-AEP): 2016 recommendations. An Pediatr (Engl Ed). 2016;84(1):60. e1-60. e13.
2. National Autonomous University of Mexico. Vaccines save lives. Revista De Divulgación Del Instituto De Biotecnología De La Unam. 2019;19.
3. Merino Moína Pediatrician El Greco Getafe Madrid MC, Bravo Acuña Pediatrician El Greco Getafe Madrid JC. Generalities about vaccines: practical things. Update Course in Pediatrics. 2018;3.
4. Galindo Santana BM, Arroyo Rojas L, Concepción Díaz D. Vaccine safety and its impact on the population. Rev Cub Salud Publica. 2011;37(1).
5. Merino Moína Pediatrician El Greco Getafe Madrid MC, Bravo Acuña Pediatrician El Greco Getafe Madrid JC. Generalities about vaccines: practical things. Update Course in Pediatrics. 2018;3.
6. WHO. Global Vaccine Action Plan. In: WHO. 2020.
7. Ministry of Health and Social Protection. What you should know about vaccines. Unicef. 2021;
8. Ricardo Gutierrez Children's Hospital. Vaccine Generalities. XV Latin American Course "Update in Immunizations at Distance 2021". 2021;
9. Aristizábal Hoyos GP, Blanco Borjas DM, Sánchez Ramos A, Ostiguín Meléndez RM. Nola Pender's model of health promotion. A reflection on its understanding. Enfermería Universitaria. 2018;8(4).
10. LatinComm. History and progress of vaccination in Mexico. LatinComm, latest review. 2015;
11. Arellán-Regalado M. Knowledge and attitudes of mothers with children under 5 years of age about vaccines. CASUS Journal of Research and Cases in Health. 2018;3(3).
12. Escobar F, Osorio M, Hoz F. Reasons for non-vaccination in children under five years of age in four Colombian cities. Pan American Journal of Public Health. 2018;41.
13. Quirola Gavilánez JC, Herrera López JL. Sociocultural factors related to compliance with vaccination schedules in children under 2 years of age during confinement. Sapienza: International Journal of Interdisciplinary Studies. 2022;3(1).
14. Auris Contreras JM. Factores Asociados En El Incumplimiento Del Calendario De Vacunacion De Los Niños Menores De 2 Años, En Un Centro De Salud-Minsa-Lima 2017. concytec. 2018;
15. Santos-Preciado JI. New vaccination schedule in Mexico. Salud Publica Mex. 1999;41(1).

16. Orellana Centeno JE, Guerrero Sotelo RN. The vaccination process in Mexico. Journal of the Mexican Dental Association. 2021;78(5).
17. Vaccination coverage in children and adolescents in Mexico: complete, incomplete and non-vaccination schedule [Internet]. [cited 2023 Mar 28]. Available from: https://www.scielo.org.mx/scielo.php?script=sci_arttext&pid=S0036-36342013000800028
18. Díaz-Ortega JL, Ferreira-Guerrero Elizabeth, Trejo-Valdivia B, Téllez-Rojo MM, Ferreyra-Reyes L, Hernández-Serrato M, et al. Vaccination coverage in children and adolescents in mexico: complete, incomplete and non-vaccination schedule. Salud Publica Mex. 2013;55(SUPPL.2).
19. Hernández-Ávila M, Palacio-Mejía LS, Hernández-Ávila JE, Charvel S. Vaccination in Mexico: imprecise coverage and deficiency in the follow-up of children who do not complete the scheme. Salud Publica Mex. 2020;62(2).
20. Repositorio Digital UCSG: Factors associated with noncompliance with the vaccination schedule in children aged 0 to 5 years belonging to a health subcenter in the city of Guayaquil. [Internet]. [cited 2023 Mar 28]. Available from: http://repositorio.ucsg.edu.ec/handle/3317/10071
21. Ricardo J, Loera-Díaz D, Nataly I, Teresa M, de Aguascalientes A, Gómez-Chávez M, et al. Reasons for noncompliance with the basic vaccination schedule in a rural community of Aguascalientes. Periodicity: Quarterly. 2021; 16:2021.
22. Ministry of Health. Specific action program for universal vaccination 2013-2018. Health Sector Program. 2018;
23. Noriega-Rubalcaba A, Nieto-Ortega E, Vivanco-Gómez E, Durán-Méndez A, Ortega DP, Peón AN. Vaccination strategy in Mexico and vaccine diversity. Revista de la Sociedad Española de Beneficencia. 2021;2(1).
24. Sociocultural factors and compliance with the national immunization schedule in children under 5 years of age at the Lliupapuquio health center - Apurimac, 2021 [Internet]. [cited 2023 Mar 28]. Available from: http://repositorio.unac.edu.pe/handle/20.500.12952/6592
25. World Health Organization. Global Vaccine Action Plan 2011-2020. World Health Organization. 2013;
26. World Health Organization. Varicella vaccines. Weekly epidemiological bulletin. 2019;87(28-29).
27. Guevara-Saldaña L, Calle-Alvarez AM, Ramirez-Giraldo RH, Chinchilla-Mejia C, Cardona-Villa R. Myths and realities about vaccine allergy. Acta Médica Colombiana. 2018;44(2).
28. Ramíres-Pereda N, Regalado-Santiago C, Cruz-Sánchez JJ, Rodríguez-Cortes O, Gonzalez Cano P. Vaccines, adjuvants and bacteriophages as vaccine vectors. BIOMEDICAL JOURNAL. 2020;31(3).

29. Galdos Kajatt O. Vaccines against human papillomavirus. Peruvian Journal of Gynecology and Obstetrics. 2018;64(3).
30. Osakidetza. Vaccination Manual. 2016. Classification of vaccines: General principles and recommendations:
31. Regalado-Vasquez ZM, Peralta-Cárdenas F, Yamasqui JL, Cruz-Gavilanes MT. Factors associated with non-compliance with the vaccination and micronutrients scheme in pregnant women of Ingapirca Parish of Cañar Canton, period November 2016-April 2017. Polo del Conocimiento. 2018;3(9).
32. Compliance with the national immunization schedule in pediatric patients attending an outpatient clinic at a tertiary level hospital [Internet]. [cited 2023 Mar 28]. Available from: https://www.imbiomed.com.mx/articulo.php?id=111093
33. Isidro Ríos TL, Gutiérrez Aguado A. Prenatal Factors Associated with Breach of The Basic Vaccination Scheme in Under 5 Years Of Age. Journal of the Faculty of Human Medicine. 2021;21(2).
34. Escobar-Díaz F, Bibiana Osorio-Merchán M, De la Hoz-Restrepo F. Reasons for non-vaccination in children under five years of age in four Colombian cities. Pan American Journal of Public Health. 2017;41.
35. Muñoz-Trinidad J, Villalobos-Navarro A, Gómez-Chávez JR, De Loera-Díaz IN, Nieto-Aguilar A, Macías-Galaviz MaT. Reasons for noncompliance with the basic vaccination schedule in a rural community of Aguascalientes. Lux Médica. 2021;16(47).
36. Medical Editorial Department of LatinComm S.A. Mexico: Pioneer country in the local production of vaccines. History and progress of vaccination in Mexico. Latest Review. 2015;
37. Di Fabio JL, Agudelo CI, Castañeda E. Regional Vaccine System (SIREVA), laboratory surveillance and vaccine development for Streptococcus pneumoniae: bibliometric analysis, 1993-2019. Pan American Journal of Public Health. 2020;44.
38. Coronada M, Hidalgo G. RNA vaccines: the most promising generation of vaccines. 2021.
39. Alarcón Velásquez LN, Mogollón Torres F de M. Adverse reactions to BCG vaccination and maternal home care in children under 1 year of age. ACC CIETNA: Journal of the School of Nursing. 2021;8(2).
40. Morales P, Balcells ME. The current relevance of BCG vaccine in the prevention of childhood tuberculosis. Andes Pediatrica. 2019;90(6).
41. Rada Cuentas J. BCG vaccine. Rev Soc Boliv Pediatr. 1998;37(1).
42. Dal Lago JE, Levy EJ. Osteomyelitis of the tibia secondary to BCG vaccination in an immunocompetent pediatric patient. Report of a case. Journal of the Argentine Association of Orthopedics and Traumatology. 2020;85(2).

43. Real Delor RE. Inadequate response to hepatitis B vaccine in health personnel of the National Hospital, Paraguay. Rev Fac Cienc Med. 2018;75(3).
44. Garassini M. Hepatitis B vaccine. Gen. 1982;36(2-3).
45. Fernández Nieto MI. Hepatitis B vaccine seroconversion in health personnel. Enfermería Investiga Investiga Investigación Vinculación Docencia y Gestión. 2019;4(3).
46. Zachou K, Sarantopoulos A, Gatselis NK, Vassiliadis T, Gabeta S, Stefos A, et al. Hepatitis B virus reactivation in hepatitis B virus surface antigen negative patients receiving immunosuppression: A hidden threat. World J Hepatol. 2013;5(7).
47. Cruchet R, Dezanet LNC, Maylin S, Gabassi A, Rougier H, Miailhes P, et al. Association of hepatitis B Core-related antigen and antihepatitis B core antibody with liver fibrosis evolution in human immunodeficiency virus-hepatitis B virus coinfected patients during treatment with tenofovir. Open Forum Infect Dis. 2020;7(7).
48. Lacruz-Rengel MA, Calderón J, Angulo F, Mata A, Quintero Y. Conocimiento materno sobre estrategias básicas de prevención en enfermedad diarreica aguda TT - Maternal knowledge of basic prevention strategies in acute diarrheal disease. Arch venez pueric pediatr. 2012;75(4).
49. Iskander JK, Gidudu J, Arboleda N, Huang WT. Selected major vaccine safety issues. Annales Nestlé (Spanish Ed). 2008;66(2).
50. González Chávez R. Seasonality of rotavirus infection in Venezuela: relationship between monthly rotavirus incidence and pluviometric indices. Invest Clin. 2015;56(3).
51. Lacruz-Rengel M, Calderón J, Angulo F, Mata A, Quintero Y. Maternal knowledge on basic prevention strategies in acute diarrheal disease. Arch Venez Pueric Pediatr. 2012;75(4).
52. Ordóñez BR. Epidemiologic investigation on the antigenic power of the anti-influenza vaccine. Prensa Med Mex. 1972;37(7).
53. Keller F. K, Sepúlveda S. O, Ibarra M. L. Equine influenza: Serological response in equines immunized with bivalent equine influenza vaccine. Advances in Veterinary Sciences. 2010;5(2).
54. Romero M, Sandoval M, Tamayo K, Vivas J, Vizcaya C, D`Apollo R. Coverage and compliance with the immunization schedule in children up to 5 years old, Las Cuibas, Lara State. Venezuelan Journal of Public Health. 2014;2(1).
55. Perret P C. Pandemic influenza one year after the first wave: What can we say now? TT - Pandemic influenza one year after the first wave: What did we learn? Revista chilena de infectología. 2010;27(2).

56. González-Abad MJ, Alonso-Sanz M. Invasive pneumococcal disease in pediatrics: what can be expected from the new 13-valent pneumococcal conjugate vaccine? Vaccines. 2012;13(3).
57. Moreno-Pérez D, Álvarez García FJ, Arístegui Fernández J, Cilleruelo Ortega MJ, Corretger Rauet JM, García Sánchez N, et al. [Immunisation schedule of the Spanish Association of Paediatrics: 2017 recommendations]. An Pediatr (Barc) [Internet]. 2017 Feb 1 [cited 2023 Mar 28];86(2):98. e1-98. e9. Available from: https://pubmed.ncbi.nlm.nih.gov/28038948/
58. Sanchez J, Ramirez R, Cardona R. Frequency of allergic reactions to MMR vaccine in patients with egg allergy. Biomedica. 2018;38(4).
59. Eduardo Mazzi Gonzales de Prada A, Aliaga Uria O, Rodrigo Diana C, Alvaraz Ivana C, Rodriguez Omar C, Cortez Victoria C, et al. Completion of the vaccination schedule in children admitted to a hospital. Vol. 47, Rev Soc Bol Ped. 2008.
60. Generalitat de Catalunya. COVID-19 Vaccine Pfizer / BioNTech. Generalitat de Catalunya Servei Català de la Salut. 2021;
61. Zhu N ZD, Wang W, Li X, Yang B, Song J. Strategies and current status of the race for SARS-CoV2 vaccine development. Nat Rev Immunol. 2019;382(7).
62. Santos ADS, Viana MCA, Chaves EMC, Bezerra ADM, Gonçalves Júnior J, Tamboril ACR. Tecnologia educacional baseada em nola pender: promoção da saúde do adolescente. Revista de Enfermagem UFPE on line. 2018;12(2).
63. Ali Y, Mekonnen FA, Molla Lakew A, Wolde HF. Poor maternal health service utilization associated with incomplete vaccination among children aged 12-23 months in Ethiopia. https://doi.org/101080/2164551520191670124 [Internet]. 2019 May 3 [cited 2023 Mar 28];16(5):1202-7. Available from: https://www.tandfonline.com/doi/abs/10.1080/21645515.2019.1670124
64. Isidro-Ríos TL, Gutiérrez-Aguado A, Prenatal Factors Associated With Noncompliance With The Basic Vaccination Scheme In Children Under Five Years Of Age. Prenatal factors associated with noncompliance with the basic vaccination schedule in children under 5 years of age. Journal of the Faculty of Human Medicine [Internet]. 2021 Mar 15 [cited 2023 Mar 28];21(2):354-63. Available from: http://www.scielo.org.pe/scielo.php?script=sci_arttext&pid=S2308-05312021000200354&lng=es&nrm=iso&tlng=es

Appendix A. Operationalization of Variables

Variable	Conceptual definition	Operational definition
Social Factors	Social factors are internal or external conditioning elements that influence people's living conditions, especially social and cultural factors.	Social factors are variables that affect mothers as a whole, both in the place and in the space where they are located, being several aspects involved, such as the degree of education, maternal occupation, accessibility and attendance to health facilities.
Cultural factors	An element or characteristic of a culture that significantly influences the development of a particular phenomenon or activity.	Constituted by the set of beliefs, knowledge and lifestyles learned, shared and transmitted within a given group, which guide the reasoning, decisions and actions of mothers in caring for their children.
Mother's commitment and self-discipline	These are the conditioning elements that contribute to achieve different results. In this case, they are causes that lead the mother to attend or not to vaccinate her children. For the World Health Organization (WHO), a factor is any circumstance or cause that induces or motivates decision making.	They are all those elements that condition an action, becoming the causes of compliance with the vaccination schedule in children under 5 years of age, according to cognitive and institutional factors, measured through a questionnaire.

Source: Cruz and Baltazar (2023)

Dependent Variables

Variable	Conceptual definition	Dimensions	Operational definition	Indicators
Socio-cultural factors (Dependent)	Socio-cultural factors are internal or external conditioning elements that influence people's living conditions, especially social and cultural factors.	Social	Social factors are variables that affect mothers as a whole, both in the place and in the space where they are located, being several aspects involved, such as the degree of education, maternal occupation, accessibility and attendance to health facilities.	Age, Educational level, Marital status, Origin, Mother tongue, Family constitution, Place of birth of the child, Number of children, Age of minor children, Occupation, Economic income, Type of housing, Transportation, Mass media advertising.
		Cultural	Constituted by the set of beliefs, knowledge and lifestyles learned, shared and transmitted within a given group, which guide mothers' reasoning, decisions and actions in caring for their children.	Customs Habits Beliefs Knowledge

Source: Cruz and Baltazar (2023)

Independent Variables

Variable	Conceptual definition	Dimensions	Operational definition	Indicators
Compliance with the National Vaccination Schedule (Independent)	These are the conditioning elements that contribute to achieve different results. In this case, they are causes that lead the mother to attend or not to vaccinate her children. For the World Health Organization (WHO), a factor is any circumstance or cause that induces or motivates decision making.	Mother's commitment Mother's self-discipline	These are all those elements that condition an action, becoming the causes of compliance with the vaccination schedule in children under 5 years of age, according to cognitive and institutional factors, measured through a questionnaire.	Commitment Time availability Attendance and continuity of appointments. Observation and dedication to child health.

Source: Cruz and Baltazar (2023)

Appendix B. Informed and Consensual Consent.

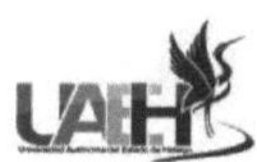

Autonomous University of the State of Hidalgo.
Pediatric Nursing Specialty.
Secretary of Research and Graduate Studies.

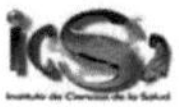

Project Title: Factors influencing non-compliance with the vaccination schedule in children from 0 to 5 years of age in a kindergarten.

Principal Author: Lic. Magda Karina Cruz García. Thesis Director: M.C.E. Rosa María Baltazar Téllez.

We invite you to participate in the research entitled "Factors that influence non-compliance with the vaccination schedule in children from 0 to 5 years of age in a kindergarten". For the realization of this research, we took into account ethical aspects based on the regulations of the General Health Law (1987) regarding the ethical aspects of research on human beings contained in the second title, chapter I and chapter III.

In Chapter I, in accordance with Article 13, the dignity and protection of the rights and welfare of the participants shall be respected.
In accordance with article 17, this was considered to be a minimal risk research in this case, since no intervention or intentional modification was performed on the physiological, psychological and social variables of the study participants.

The information that Ms. Magda Karina Cruz García obtains from this interview will be used for the completion of her Thesis as a requirement for the Postgraduate Degree in Pediatric Nursing at the Universidad Autónoma del Estado de Hidalgo.

Your participation will consist of giving me a survey, which will last 20 minutes. The information you provide will be kept under the protection of the researchers. The anonymity of your name will be protected by using numbers and codes to classify the surveys.
Your participation is voluntary, which means that you should not feel pressured to participate for any reason, and you will not receive any financial incentive for your participation. If you wish, you have the right to refuse to participate and to withdraw from the study at any time. This decision will be respected. (Ethical principle number 8.- Although the main objective of medical research is to generate new knowledge, this objective should never take precedence over the rights and interests of the person participating in the research).

I____ have been invited to participate in the research "Factors influencing non-compliance with the vaccination schedule in children from 0 to 5 years old in a kindergarten".

My participation will be through a survey:

I have read the information

2. I have had the opportunity to ask questions and these have been answered satisfactorily.
3. I voluntarily agree to participate in the research, and I understand the right to withdraw at any time from the study, without being affected in any way.

Participant's name: ________________________________

Mother's Name: ___________________________________

Signature: ____

Annex C. Evaluation Instrument

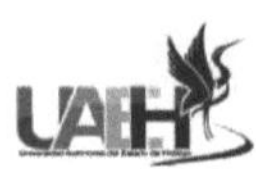

Autonomous University of the State of Hidalgo.
Pediatric Nursing Specialty.
Secretary of Research and Graduate Studies.

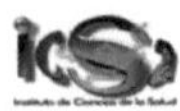

"Evaluation questionnaire to identify sociocultural factors and their relationship to compliance with the national immunization schedule in children under 5 years of age"
CEIFSRCENVNMA (2023).

Dear Madam, the purpose of this questionnaire is to obtain information on the sociocultural factors that influence compliance with the vaccination schedule, for which your collaboration is sincerely requested; expressing that it is anonymous. The data you provide will be confidential and anonymous.

INSTRUCTIONS: Mark with an (X) the option you consider correct, choose only one alternative. Do not leave questions blank. Thank you.

SOCIAL FACTORS

Age:

a. 19 or less
b. from 20 to 30
c. from 31 to 40
d. over 41 years old

2.- What is your marital status?

a. single
b. married
c. free union
d. divorced
e. widower

3.- Occupation:

a. student
b. housewife
c. private employee
d. public employee

4.- Level of study:

a. illiterate
b. primary
c. secondary
d. bachelor's degree
e. postgraduate

5.- Mother's origin

a. Colony
b. Sierra
c. Municipality
d. City

6.- Mother tongue:

a. Spanish

b. English
c. Indigenous language

7.- Your family is composed of:

a. dad, mom, and kids
b. mom and kids
c. father and children
d. mom or dad, children and grandparents

8.- Place of birth of the child:

a. Clinic
b. Hospital
c. Health center
d. At home

9.- How many children do you have?

a. less than 3
b. 3 or 4 children
c. 5 or 6 children
d. 7 children or more

10.- Age of the minor child:

a. 7 months or less
b. from 8 to 15 months
c. from 16 to 23 months
d. from 2 to 5 years old

11.- What is your monthly family income?

a. greater than $4900
b. from $2000 to $4800
c. less than $2000
d. no income

12.- The house you live in is:

a. Own
b. Family
c. Rented
d. borrowed

13.- What means of transportation do you use to take your child to get vaccinated?

a. private transportation
b. cab
c. bus
d. on foot

14.- Have you heard any publicity regarding the type of vaccination your child usually receives? a. Always

b. Sometimes
c. Very seldom
d. Never

CULTURAL FACTORS

15.- In your family, do you usually take your children to be vaccinated?

a. Always
b. Sometimes
c. Very seldom
d. Never

16.- Do you consider that receiving several vaccines simultaneously weakens the immune system?
a. always
b. Sometimes
c. Very seldom
d. Never

17.- If other people advise you not to vaccinate your child, would you take him/her to be vaccinated?

a. always
b. Sometimes
c. Very seldom
d. Never

18.- In case your children present fever, diarrhea, cold or are under treatment, would you take them to be vaccinated?

a. Takes him to the pediatrician
b. Gives remedy
c. I would vaccinate again
d. You would make your discomfort known

19.- Do you believe that vaccines are necessary and why?

a. Prevent or protect against serious diseases.
b. They are medicines to cure diseases.
c. Aids in their proper growth and development.
d. Unknown

20.- In the event that your child misses his/her immunization appointment; do you consider that:

a. It is necessary to continue
b. no need to continue
c. should look like this
d. unknown

21.- Do you think it is necessary to give the child booster vaccines?

a. Always
b. Sometimes
c. Very seldom
d. Never

22.- Can homemade medicines replace vaccines?

a. Always
b. Sometimes
c. Very seldom
d. Never

23.- Do you consider that vaccines are dangerous and harmful to health?

a. Always
b. Sometimes
c. Very seldom
d. Never

COMPLIANCE WITH THE VACCINATION CARD

24.- Have you so far complied with your children's immunization schedule?
- a. Always
- b. Sometimes
- c. Very seldom
- d. Never

25.- Do you feel committed to keep your vaccination appointments?
- a. Always
- b. Sometimes
- c. Very seldom
- d. Never

26.- Do you feel committed to informing yourself about the benefits of vaccines?
- a. Always
- b. Sometimes
- c. Very seldom
- d. Never

27.- Do you have the time to attend your child's immunization appointments?
- a. Always
- b. Sometimes
- c. Very seldom
- d. Never

28.- Would you entrust the vaccination of your child to a very trusted relative?
- a. Always
- b. Sometimes
- c. Very seldom
- d. Never

29.- Can homemade medicines replace vaccines?
- a. Always
- b. Sometimes
- c. Very seldom
- d. Never

30.- if a vaccine cannot be fulfilled, do you look for a way to find a solution?
- a. Always
- b. Sometimes
- c. Very seldom
- d. Never

MOTHER'S SELF-DISCIPLINE

31.- Do you attend scheduled appointments?
- a. Always
- b. Sometimes
- c. Very seldom
- d. Never

Do you maintain continuity in the vaccination schedule?
- a. Always
- b. Sometimes
- c. Very seldom
- d. Never

33.- Do you consider that vaccines are dangerous and harmful to health?
- a. Always

b. Sometimes
c. Very seldom
d. Never

34.- Do you keep track of monthly or annual vaccination appointments in addition to the vaccination card?

a. Always
b. Sometimes
c. Very seldom
d. Never

35.- Do you think it is necessary to give the child several vaccines at the same time?

a. Always
b. Sometimes
c. Very seldom
d. Never

36.- If your child presents any disease other than the symptoms of the vaccines, would you blame it on the vaccines?

a. Always
b. Sometimes
c. Very seldom
d. Never

37.- Do you self-medicate your child?

a. Always
b. Sometimes
c. Very seldom
d. Never

38.- What is the main reason you missed your vaccination appointment?

a. Can't remember the date
b. Loss of card
c. Lack of time
d. Difficulty in getting to the Health Center.

¡¡¡¡¡Thank you for your participation!!!!

Exhibit D. Research Authorization

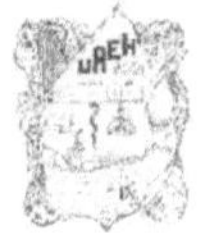

UNIVERSIDAD AUTÓNOMA DEL ESTADO DE HIDALGO
Instituto de Ciencias de la Salud
Área Académica de Enfermería

14/abril/2023

Of. Núm. 015

Asunto: Autorización de investigación

MTRA. SANDY CORONA GREZ
DIRECTORA DEL JARDIN DE NIÑOS JOSE VASCONCELOS
SAN JUAN TIZAHUAPAN, EPAZOTUCAN, HIDALGO

Por medio del presente me permito, solicitar su autorización para que la estudiante del Posgrado en Enfermería Pediátrica de la Universidad Autónoma del Estado de Hidalgo, L. E. Magda Karina Cruz García aplique su protocolo de investigación titulado "Factores que influyen el incumplimiento en el esquema de vacunación en niños escolares", toda a vez que ella se encuentra realizando su tesis para su obtención de grado como enfermera especialista en pediatría, haciendo mención que este proyecto esta asesorado por una investigadora experta en el área, y la información que se recabará solamente será utilizada para los fines académicos de la interesada, y en lo que se apega a la Ley General de Salud en materia de investigación, se les otorgará previamente a los participantes y padres de familia y/o tutores un consentimiento informado y consensuado. Para validar la autorización en la participación de este estudio. Cabe hacer mención que las fechas que se utilizarán son los días 19, 20 y 21 del presente mes en un horario de 9:00 am a 12:00 pm.

Sin más por el momento, esperando sea favorecido con su gentil y valioso apoyo le envió un cordial saludo.

ATENTAMENTE
"AMOR, ORDEN Y PROGRESO"

M.C.E. ROSA MARIA BALTAZAR TÉLLEZ
COORDINADORA DE LA ESPECIALIDAD EN ENFERMERIA PEDIATRICA

EDUCACIÓN
SECRETARÍA DE EDUCACIÓN PÚBLICA
DIRECCIÓN DE EDUCACIÓN PREESCOLAR GENERAL
SUPERVISIÓN ZONA 93
JARDÍN DE NIÑOS "JOSÉ VASCONCELOS"
C.C.T. 13DJN0463S
CALLE EL JIRÓN ESQ. NIÑO PERDIDO
SAN JUAN TIZAHUAPAN, MPIO. EPAZOYUCAN, HGO.

Recibí original 17/04/23

C.C.P. INTERESADO

www.uaeh.edu.mx

Exhibit E. Application Authorization

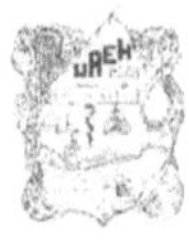

UNIVERSIDAD AUTÓNOMA DEL ESTADO DE HIDALGO
Instituto de Ciencias de la Salud
Área Académica de Enfermería

14/abril/2023
Of. Núm. 015
Asunto: Autorización de investigación

MTRA. SANDY CORONA GREZ
DIRECTORA DEL JARDIN DE NIÑOS JOSE VASCONCELOS
SAN JUAN TIZAHUAPAN, EPAZOTUCAN, HIDALGO

Por medio del presente me permito, solicitar su autorización para que la estudiante del Posgrado en Enfermería Pediátrica de la Universidad Autónoma del Estado de Hidalgo, L. E. Magda Karina Cruz García aplique su protocolo de investigación titulado "Factores que influyen el incumplimiento en el esquema de vacunación en niños escolares", toda a vez que ella se encuentra realizando su tesis para su obtención de grado como enfermera especialista en pediatría, haciendo mención que este proyecto esta asesorado por una investigadora experta en el área, y la información que se recabará solamente será utilizada para los fines académicos de la interesada, y en lo que se apega a la Ley General de Salud en materia de investigación, se les otorgará previamente a los participantes y padres de familia y/o tutores un consentimiento informado y consensuado. Para validar la autorización en la participación de este estudio. Cabe hacer mención que las fechas que se utilizarán son los días 19, 20 y 21 del presente mes en un horario de 9:00 am a 12:00 pm.

Sin más por el momento, esperando sea favorecido con su gentil y valioso apoyo le envió un cordial saludo.

ATENTAMENTE
"AMOR, ORDEN Y PROGRESO"

M.C.E. ROSA MARIA BALTAZAR TÉLLEZ
COORDINADORA DE LA ESPECIALIDAD EN ENFERMERIA PEDIATRICA

EDUCACIÓN
SECRETARÍA DE EDUCACIÓN PÚBLICA
DIRECCIÓN DE EDUCACIÓN PREESCOLAR GENERAL
SUPERVISIÓN ZONA 93
JARDÍN DE NIÑOS "JOSÉ VASCONCELOS"
C.C.T. 13DJN0453S
CALLE EL JIRÓN ESQ. NIÑO PERDIDO SAN JUAN TIZAHUAPAN, MPIO. EPAZOYUCAN, HGO.

Recibí original 17/04/23

C.C.P. INTERESADO

www.uaeh.edu.mx

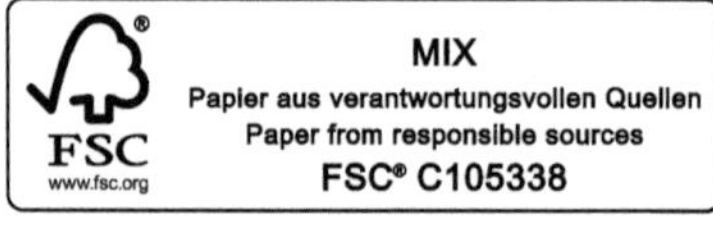

Printed by Books on Demand GmbH, Norderstedt / Germany